Cambridge Elements ≡

Elements of Improving Quality and Safety in Healthcare
edited by
Mary Dixon-Woods,* Katrina Brown,* Sonja Marjanovic,†
Tom Ling,† Ellen Perry,* Graham Martin,* Gemma Petley,* and
Claire Dipple*
*THIS Institute (The Healthcare Improvement Studies Institute)
†RAND Europe

SUPPLY CHAIN
MANAGEMENT

Sharon J. Williams
School of Health and Social Care, Swansea University

THIS.Institute The Healthcare Improvement Studies Institute

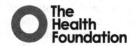

CAMBRIDGE
UNIVERSITY PRESS

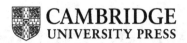

Shaftesbury Road, Cambridge CB2 8EA, United Kingdom

One Liberty Plaza, 20th Floor, New York, NY 10006, USA

477 Williamstown Road, Port Melbourne, VIC 3207, Australia

314–321, 3rd Floor, Plot 3, Splendor Forum, Jasola District Centre,
New Delhi – 110025, India

103 Penang Road, #05–06/07, Visioncrest Commercial, Singapore 238467

Cambridge University Press is part of Cambridge University Press & Assessment,
a department of the University of Cambridge.

We share the University's mission to contribute to society through the pursuit of
education, learning and research at the highest international levels of excellence.

www.cambridge.org
Information on this title: www.cambridge.org/9781009325288

DOI: 10.1017/9781009325271

First published 2024

A catalogue record for this publication is available from the British Library.

ISBN 978-1-009-32528-8 Paperback
ISSN 2754-2912 (online)
ISSN 2754-2904 (print)

Cambridge University Press & Assessment has no responsibility for the persistence
or accuracy of URLs for external or third-party internet websites referred to in this
publication and does not guarantee that any content on such websites is, or will
remain, accurate or appropriate.

Every effort has been made in preparing this Element to provide accurate and
up-to-date information that is in accord with accepted standards and practice at the
time of publication. Although case histories are drawn from actual cases, every effort
has been made to disguise the identities of the individuals involved. Nevertheless, the
authors, editors, and publishers can make no warranties that the information
contained herein is totally free from error, not least because clinical standards are
constantly changing through research and regulation. The authors, editors, and
publishers therefore disclaim all liability for direct or consequential damages resulting
from the use of material contained in this Element. Readers are strongly advised to pay
careful attention to information provided by the manufacturer of any drugs or
equipment that they plan to use.

Supply Chain Management

Elements of Improving Quality and Safety in Healthcare

DOI: 10.1017/9781009325271
First published online: November 2024

Sharon J. Williams
School of Health and Social Care, Swansea University
Author for correspondence: Sharon J. Williams,
sharon.j.williams@swansea.ac.uk

Abstract: Creating a well-integrated, resilient, and highly transparent supply chain is central to effective and safe patient care. But managing healthcare supply chains is complex; common challenges include the underuse, overuse, and misuse of health resources. This Element introduces the key principles and definitions of healthcare supply chains. Practical insights into the design and operation of healthcare supply chains are provided. Core characteristics of effective supply chain management such as performance management, systems thinking, and supply chain integration are examined along with the application of specific supply chain design and improvement approaches. Finally, the Element proposes areas that require further development both in research and practice. This title is also available as Open Access on Cambridge Core.

Keywords: supply chain, supplier networks, supply chain management, supply chain integration, systems thinking

ISBNs: 9781009325288 (PB), 9781009325271 (OC)
ISSNs: 2754-2912 (online), 2754-2904 (print)

Contents

1 Introduction

Well-integrated, resilient, and highly transparent supply chains that are responsive to the needs of health systems and patients are essential to quality and safety, but they are vulnerable to complex operational management problems.[1–6] Healthcare settings carry large quantities of items that may be very diverse, ranging from pharmaceuticals, surgical medical products, medical equipment, and sterile items through to linen and food. Supply chain management (SCM) is needed to distribute supplies to point-of-care locations, handle physical goods, and manage the flow of patients.[7] Good SCM can lead to reduced cycle times (time taken to complete a process from start to finish), lower organisational costs, and better performance without compromising quality.[8] By contrast, poor understanding and management of supply chains can result in suboptimal performance,[9] including supply bottlenecks, short-term demand fluctuations, and inappropriate ad hoc purchasing decisions. However, until the COVID-19 pandemic, healthcare has not always given SCM the attention it deserves.[10,11] Pandemic-related global shortages of medical products highlighted the vulnerability of medical product supply chains,[12,13] demonstrating the need for supply chains that are resilient and responsive, and the systemic risks they face.[12,14] Accordingly, SCM emphasising good service delivery, patient safety, and cost control[15] is an important, if sometimes neglected, improvement approach in healthcare.[3]

Supply chain management is complex, involving many different flows of activities, functions, and multiple stakeholders.[16,17] It has been researched within many different disciplines, including marketing, logistics, economics, and systems dynamics.[18] The range of disciplines involved means that no single agreed definition of SCM has emerged. Instead, SCM is a term widely used to mean somewhat different things depending on role, specialism, or discipline. Its value as a catch-all phrase is that it includes multiple aspects of procurement, logistics, operations, technology, and facilities management. These often operate at a national or global scale and are all relevant to high-quality patient care processes.

This Element begins by introducing the key principles and definitions of healthcare supply chains. It provides a practical insight into their design and operation, covering health services, pharmaceutical, specialist services, and humanitarian services supply chains. This is followed by an exploration of the core characteristics of effective SCM such as performance management, systems thinking, and supply chain integration. The application of specific supply chain design and improvement approaches such as Lean and Agile is discussed. A critique of the application of SCM in healthcare is provided, and areas of further development identified.

2 Principles and Definitions

A supply chain can be defined as a 'network of organizations that are involved, through upstream and downstream linkages, in the different processes and activities that produce value in the form of products and services in the hands of the ultimate consumer'.[19] Supply chain management has been a popular concept in industry since the 1990s, when Christopher[20] recognised that competition was no longer about companies competing against each other, but about the performance of entire supply chains. Organisations are increasingly concerned not only to improve their own performance, but also to be active in the development of their immediate suppliers (known as first-tier suppliers), their suppliers' suppliers (second-tier suppliers), and so on.

Some high-profile examples illustrate the impact of highly effective and efficient supply chains. Amazon manages a large assortment of products and offers quick deliveries at competitive prices.[21] The fashion chain Zara compresses the product design-production-delivery cycle to 15 days to rapidly replenish stock in response to customer demand.[22] Analyses attribute the operational and financial success of these ventures to a holistic approach to SCM, supported by a well-integrated information system that facilitates rapid data feedback from all parts of the supply chain.[21,22]

In healthcare, we can think of supply chains as the connection of those involved in delivering the care that a patient needs.[23] De Vries and Huijsman[10] suggest that healthcare SCM covers the management of people, processes, information, and finances to deliver products and services, enabling the flow of patients through the care system while enhancing clinical outcomes and user experience and controlling costs.[24]

Healthcare supply chains can be understood as a network formation where organisations are involved, through 'upstream' (supply) and 'downstream' (distribution) linkages, in the different processes and activities from pre-diagnosis through to post-diagnosis and possibly ongoing care. As Figure 1 shows, we can also differentiate between an internal and external supply chain. An internal supply chain operates within an organisation – for example, the distribution of medicines, materials, and equipment within operating theatres, emergency departments, and wards. An external supply chain refers to a network of providers of products and services that are external to the organisation – for example, manufacturers and distributors of medical equipment and their agents.

Both descriptions tend to suggest a linear arrangement in which patients, information, and materials all flow in one direction. But it may not work that way in practice – especially for patients with complex conditions who rely on a network of professionals, providers, and resources to deliver their care.

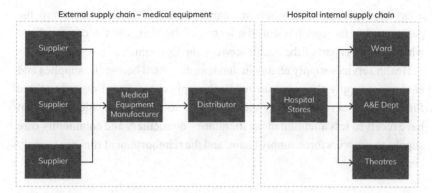

Figure 1 An internal and external medical equipment supply chain

3 Healthcare Supply Chains in Practice

In Section 2, we distinguished between the internal and external supply chain, while recognising that SCM is not always linear and often involves a network of organisations and providers. Healthcare supply chains can be classified in various ways. Betcheva et al.[24] have categorised four key areas:

- health services supply chains
- pharmaceutical supply chains
- special health services supply chains
- humanitarian supply chains in healthcare.

In this section, we examine each category in turn and identify some of the challenges and opportunities within each. Some of these supply chains have received more attention than others, partly due to maturity of supply chain practice in the more 'product based' supply chains (e.g. equipment, pharmaceutical). Other supply chains relating, for example, to patient flows and financial flows have received less attention and our understanding of these continues to develop.

3.1 Health Services Supply Chains

The number of organisations involved in the delivery of healthcare services, or a specific patient pathway depends partly on the health condition and how it is managed. That process may start and end with the same healthcare provider organisation, or it may involve multiple participants and organisations and several supply chains. Collecting information from and about the patient usually happens before the supply of services, since patients typically go through an administrative and bureaucratic process (e.g. to make an appointment or attend a service) before meeting a healthcare professional. Everything from how the patient makes the appointment, the length of the wait, and the comfort level while waiting is part of the health services supply chain.

Health services supply chains include, as discussed below, the supplies and equipment supply chain and the medical supply chain. Box 1 describes three further health services supply chains crucial to delivering patient care that have received less attention in the literature – domiciliary and community care supply chain, workforce supply chain, and the reimbursement (finance) supply chain.

3.1.1 Supplies and Equipment Supply Chain

The crucially important supplies and equipment[24] supply chain typically starts with the manufacturer and ends with the healthcare provider (see Figure 2). Depending on what is being purchased, some are delivered directly to the provider and others will be routed via distributors, agencies, or logistic providers. Consumables and non-specialist items are often procured by national purchasing organisations. In hospitals, products then need to be distributed via the internal stores.

Much of the research in this area focuses on flows of supplies and material within an internal supply chain (e.g. how these supplies are managed within a hospital) or dyadic (two party) relations between hospitals and their supplier, rather than on the entire supply chain network. The focus is largely on reducing inventory, improving stock management (by limiting shortages and obsolete stock), and increasing communication (see, for example, Kelle et al.[25]).

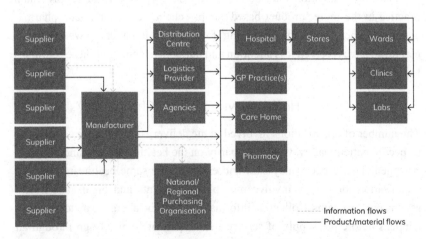

Figure 2 A healthcare supply chain for supplies and equipment

BOX 1 ADDITIONAL EXAMPLES OF HEALTH SERVICE SUPPLY CHAINS

Community and Social Care Supply Chain

The community and social care supply chain relates to home and residential care provided within communities. This covers a wide range of services, including district nursing, health promotion, and therapy services. These services are often provided to patients with complex needs and long-term conditions. Key stakeholders within the supply chain are local authorities, social services, and providers of residential and home care along with care provided by families and friends. Providers of care also extend to the private sector. The increasing demand on both health and social care requires a well-aligned and integrated supply chain that focuses on the delivery of patient-centred care.[24]

Workforce Supply Chain

The workforce supply chain focuses on the education and provision of health and social care staff. Key stakeholders include educational institutions, professional bodies, and policy-makers. Healthcare professionals – healthcare scientists, nurses, pharmacists, doctors, therapists, and mission-critical staff including managers, healthcare assistants, and cleaning and catering personnel – are vital to the provision of care. Despite the introduction of new roles such as advanced nurse practitioners, workforce shortages are still common across health and social care. Clearly, this has a negative impact on patient care and staff well-being.[28] If the gap between the number of staff working in the health and care system and the number of staff needed to meet demand continues to grow, then the quality of care will deteriorate, and patient safety risks will increase.[29] Redesigning key processes such as workforce planning and recruitment can help reduce delays and duplication in what have often become lengthy and bureaucratic parts of the workforce supply chain.

Reimbursement Supply Chain

The reimbursement (finance) supply chain is also a key part of the health services supply chain. Referring to financial flows and various reimbursement models, these supply chains are highly variable across different countries (see the Element on health economics[30]). Payment systems are often complicated, department or specialist-based, and not well coordinated or integrated across care pathways. This may limit cooperative and collaborative behaviour and integration across different providers of care. Possibly due to the myriad of local and national financial systems operating within healthcare networks, few studies have attempted to map and improve financial flows.

3.1.2 Medical Supply Chain

What Betcheva et al.[24] refer to as the medical supply chain encompasses the patient journey from the first point of contact, often the general practitioner (GP), through to secondary care in a hospital or clinic, and tertiary or highly specialised care, such as cancer treatment. Process mapping is often used to capture a high-level understanding of the patient journey via the different services within this supply chain (see Figure 3 and other examples[24,26,27]). Issues that can arise in the medical supply chain include delayed transfer of patients from emergency department to the ward and then delayed discharge to home or other services. Betcheva et al.[24] suggest that these are often the result of fragmented and poorly coordinated supply chains, filled with uncertainty.[24]

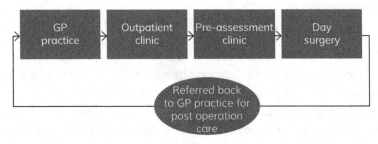

Figure 3 A high-level medical supply chain for day surgery

3.2 Pharmaceutical Supply Chains

The pharmaceutical supply chain is a good example of healthcare interacting with manufacturing and distribution supply chains. Generally comprising a 'combination of processes, organisations and operations involved in the development, design and manufacturing of useful pharmaceutical drugs',[31] it is reported to be one of the most complex supply chains. This is because it relates to the life and the health of individuals and involves high levels of risk, uncertainty, and significant irregularity in information flows throughout the chain.[32] Typically, it brings together many different stakeholders – including raw material producers, manufacturers, wholesalers and distributors, pharmacies and healthcare providers, healthcare professionals, and patients[33,34] – often with diverse and competing objectives.

Standard areas of SCM, such as facility location, capacity planning, production planning, inventory management, and scheduling all play crucial roles in managing pharmaceutical supply chains. Other factors specific to the pharmaceutical industry, such as inventory management of perishable pharmaceuticals and price competition controlled by a small number of companies, necessitate the need for a well-managed and integrated supply chain that optimises transparency and performance.[35] The need is further amplified by changes the global pharmaceutical industry has gone through in the past decade, many relating to the adoption of new technologies. It is increasingly having to address challenges relating to counterfeit drugs[36] and operational issues, including cold chains (for vaccines and medicines requiring storage at low temperature), and the security of logistics and transportation.

3.2.1 Vaccine Supply Chain

Vaccine supply chains have recently been the focus of increased attention. The preventative vaccine supply chain, which includes influenza and childhood immunisation programmes, is well established. Reactive vaccinations may also be needed during an infectious disease outbreak, as seen in the COVID-19 pandemic. Successful vaccination campaigns rely on good logistics and SCM.[37] Accordingly, the World Health Organization[38] provides guidance for countries to develop and strengthen their supply chain strategies to order, receive, store, distribute, and manage COVID-19 vaccines and their ancillary products. Advice also includes cold chain and logistic requirements, security, waste management, and reverse logistics (managing the end-of-use and end-of-life of products and equipment), along with a self-assessment SCM readiness checklist.

A literature review conducted before the pandemic identifies four key components in the vaccine supply chain.[37] First is the decision on which product to use, as multiple vaccinations may be available for the same disease. Policy-makers must also decide how the vaccines are to be scheduled, delivered, and stored. Second, decisions on vaccine production are dogged by uncertainty in terms of quantities and lead times, but collaboration between key stakeholders can improve the match between demand and supply. Third is allocation of the vaccine. This is another key decision, as usually there are insufficient quantities to vaccinate the entire population, especially in the case of sudden outbreaks such as COVID-19. The final step is the distribution of vaccines from the manufacturer to the end user, which needs to be carefully managed in terms of logistics, storage, inventory management, and staffing levels to administer the vaccines.

The review concludes that the vaccine supply chain has two distinctive characteristics. First is the misalignment of objectives and decentralised decision-making, with many involved stakeholders having competing interests. The second is the quantitative difference between low-income and high-income countries. This difference is most apparent in the distribution phase. Since most vaccines need to be stored at low temperatures, reliable electricity systems to provide refrigeration are crucial. Unfortunately, such reliable systems are not available in many developing countries. Events such as plant failures, contamination problems, epidemiological outbreaks, earthquakes, and wars may also have a serious impact on the vaccine supply chain.[39] Interestingly, most studies focus on the production of vaccines for seasonal influenza; prior to the COVID-19 pandemic, very few studies took an SCM perspective on the production of vaccines for sudden outbreaks.[37]

Box 2 outlines two other health services supply chains – the blood supply chain and the organ transplantation supply chain – both interfacing with health services supply chains (Section 3.1) and, to some extent, pharmaceutical supply chains.

Box 2 Special supply chains

Blood Supply Chain

The blood supply chain is a specialist and complex network of donors and organisations involved in the storage, testing, and distribution of blood products.[40] Starting with the donation of blood at dedicated facilities, blood units are then transported, processed, and stored at blood banks before being distributed to hospitals and administered to patients. The supply of donor blood is irregular, and demand is difficult to predict and further complicated by the perishability of blood products. Shortages can cause an increase in mortality rate, but maintaining supply is challenged by mandatory time intervals between donations.

Organ Donation and Transplantation Supply Chain

The organ donation and transplantation supply chain has received limited attention within the supply chain literature. This is surprising given the need to manage and coordinate various stakeholders and processes within a limited time. Not only are donors scarce, but organ losses can and do occur. Research has examined the process of donation, organ retrieval, and the transplantation procedure itself with inadequate logistics (storage, transport, and handling) reported as one of the causes of donation failures. Multimodality (joint use of helicopters, airplanes, drones, and emergency vehicles) is suggested to optimise transportation of organs.[41]

3.3 Humanitarian Supply Chains in Healthcare

A growing literature focuses on humanitarian supply chains. Typically, these involve government donors, international agencies, international and local non-governmental organisations, local partners, and aid recipients.[42] Bhattacharya et al.[43] and Holguín-Veras et al.[44] highlight differences in design requirements and coordination mechanisms between humanitarian and traditional supply chains. Humanitarian supply chains are often unstable and cover a wide range of operational conditions, spanning different forms of humanitarian assistance – from those set in relatively stable environments over a sustained period of time to more chaotic and dynamic post-disaster environments.[44] Often relief efforts are compromised due to lack of visibility, limited or absent information sharing, mistrust among disaster relief workers, and poor collaboration among agencies.[45,46] The humanitarian supply chain therefore has to be agile and responsive to the changing needs of end users through an effective information infrastructure and through sensitive needs assessment at field level.[42]

Collaboration and coordination across the supply chain is required to manage multi-facility and multi-supplier networks and the challenges that aid agencies face in disaster relief operations.[47] Coordination of resources (human resources, equipment, and goods) is impacted by the unpredictability of demand and uncontrollable environmental factors. Public health issues and refugee well-being are central to any humanitarian supply chain activity, so being able to provide health treatments, strategies, and solutions to combat diseases in refugee camps are critical and a high priority. Previous research suggests a lack of process standardisation for certain types of operations, both within and across different humanitarian organisations, and of common templates to facilitate the interoperability between humanitarian organisations in areas such as needs assessment, ordering, and tracking items.[47,48] There is also a demand for targeted local logistics training and education.[48,49]

4 Improving Healthcare Supply Chains

Supply chain management is key to reducing waste, increasing productivity and material flow, improving quality, and reducing costs.[50] It seeks to improve operational efficiency while enhancing responsiveness to customers, so supply chain principles call for optimising processes and operations throughout the supply chain network to improve quality and control costs.[9] Timely access to supplies, for example, helps to make best use of scarce resources and manage the flow of patients. For material flows, inventory insight and visibility can provide real-time data to make informed decisions and help to manage inventory at a faster pace, update replenishment systems, and improve overall performance of the supply chain.

However, managing healthcare supply chains is challenging and the skills to do so remain scarce, to the extent that SCM is sometimes mistakenly assumed to be limited to procurement.[9] Betcheva et al.[51] identify four categories of challenges associated with the management of healthcare supply chains:

- clinical and public health issues, for example, uncertainty of disease/prognosis, medical errors
- operational issues such as third-party finances, unclear performance measures
- fragmented care, for example, siloed working and lack of coordinated care
- financial issues often relating to the complexity of payment systems.

These challenges emphasise the need to take a systems approach to SCM that spans across a multitude of stakeholders to reflect the entire patient journey. While this is complex, greater understanding of the design and performance of these supply chains can support improvement.

In this section, we outline the key characteristics and capabilities of supply chains, followed by the important role of managing logistics. We also examine supply chain design by considering how concepts such as Lean, Agile, and Leagility have been applied within healthcare to improve performance. This is followed by a discussion of managing and improving patient flow which continues to attract considerable attention both in relation to individual (e.g. hospital) supply chains and the wider healthcare system. Then, we consider the advances in technology and the humanistic points of culture and supply chain expertise. Where possible examples are drawn from the various types of supply chains introduced in Section 3.

4.1 Essential Core Characteristics for Effective SCM

Supply chain strategies and organisational alignment, performance management systems, systems thinking, and supply chain integration are essential characteristics of effective SCM.

4.1.1 Supply Chain Strategies and Organisational Alignment

A well-defined supply chain strategy is fundamental for managing and aligning internal and external supply chain processes and controlling supply chain costs. Key elements of supply chain strategy described in the extensive literature in this area include:

- describing clearly what customers/patients need and value
- conducting an internal assessment of supply chain capabilities (e.g. benchmarking)
- examining service and industry trends
- assessing the use of evolving technologies

- identifying and managing any potential risks or expected changes in the way that services will be delivered.

It is clear from the literature that an effective strategy needs to start with understanding how supply chains are currently performing and align with the overall strategy of an organisation. Organisations also need to consider the nature of the services or products they provide, the resources and capabilities they have, and the environment in which they operate.[51]

4.1.2 Performance Management Systems

Measuring the performance of the supply chain is fundamental to identifying and addressing any deficiencies and is a key step in maintaining and improving quality. Performance management covers activities such as defining, planning, measuring, monitoring, and improving a system's performance. Several frameworks – such as the Balanced Scorecard (BSC)[52] and the Supply Chain Operations Reference (SCOR) model (originally developed by the Supply Chain Council to be used across industries/sectors)[53] – provide an integrated performance measurement system for managing healthcare supply chains. These can be used to take a holistic approach to performance measures and to improve and communicate SCM activities within and between all supply chain members. SCOR, for example, measures against five performance attributes: reliability, responsiveness, agility, costs, and asset management efficiency. Organisations can use these to define supply chain processes, assess which performance attributes to prioritise, and identify areas that need to be improved.[54]

An adapted list of key performance measures for an internal supply chain that focuses mainly on managing inventory is set out in Box 3.[55]

4.1.3 Systems Thinking and Supply Chain Integration

Supply chain management research generally, but particularly in manufacturing, has identified a move away from simple transactions and contract-based relationships towards longer term relationships of coordination and collaboration between supply chain members. This integration of suppliers and providers is one of the key elements of SCM, and it aims to enhance and align operational and strategic capabilities of participants to improve the performance of the entire supply chain network.[56] The defining characteristics of seamless supplier-provider integration are good coordination, clear schedules, integrated processes, shared information, shared technology, long-term contracts, better quality improvement, improved supplier capability, and shared risks and rewards.

BOX 3 ADAPTED LIST OF KEY PERFORMANCE MEASURES FOR AN INTERNAL SUPPLY CHAIN
FOCUSING ON MANAGING INVENTORY

Quality
- availability of stock (e.g. no stock available, service levels)
- inventory visibility (e.g. safety stock – held in inventory to reduce risk of no stock)
- how critical inventory items are
- patient safety (e.g. delays, errors).

Time
- replenishment
- clinical staff involvement.

Finance
- inventory cost
- value of stock
- stock wastage
- total acquisition cost.

Productivity
- inventory turnover
- utilisation rates.

This movement towards integration may be seen as the innovative adaptation of the principle of 'swift and even flow'[57] in pursuit of a 'seamless supply chain'.[58] Systems thinking allows consideration of the whole rather than discrete, individual elements[59] and treats such problems as being the result of interactions across the system (supply chain) rather than the result of a single, broken component. Long-term, close collaboration based on SCM principles tends to reduce transaction costs both internally (e.g. drawing up service level agreements) and externally (e.g. undertaking market reviews and managing contracts) as well as decreasing review/inspection costs among supply chain members. Achieving a reduction in costs without compromising quality requires collaborative work with supply chain members to review activities and associated costs and eliminate activities that don't add value. This contributes to improved performance and increased profitability for the entire supply chain.

But the way healthcare is structured and delivered can have a profound effect on efficiency and effectiveness of supply chains. Earlier we noted the complexity around the reimbursement supply chain and the financial flows more generally. Budgetary controls across the healthcare system often discourage collaboration and risk further fragmentation of processes and poorly coordinated care across various providers, such as health and social care.[51] A 'functional and/or clinical silo' mentality and 'turf protection' attitudes can inhibit attempts to improve healthcare systems[60] and are sometimes, at least in part, a response to changing policies and approaches to performance measurement and budgetary reforms that focus on individual providers and suppliers.[61] Further, Coleman and Jennings[62] make the interesting observation that healthcare supply chain members consider the 'pie' (profit) as being fixed, which results in antagonistic negotiation behaviour and a focus of effort on containing (i.e. lowering) the acquisition price of supplies and services, instead of seeking to lower the *total* delivered cost. Managers could instead support and improve the performance of their supply chain members and try to increase the 'profit' for everyone involved.

4.2 Managing Logistics in Healthcare

How logistics are managed in healthcare lags behind industry and is regarded as a priority target for improvement.[63] Transportation and inventory costs are a major component of supply chain costs. According to Doone,[64] for example, the warehousing of medical devices has been fraught with waste and inefficiency. Warehouses may only be 60–70 per cent full at any given time, yet 100 per cent of the infrastructure cost must be maintained. Another key indicator is stock/inventory turns, which is the number of times inventory is sold or used within a specific time period such as a year. For medical devices this is reported to be 2, whereas in consumer electronics it is 44, in the automotive industry it is 10, and in consumer packaging 6.[64]

Use of logistics tools such as vendor management inventory (VMI) can reduce supply chain costs. With VMI, the manufacturer is responsible for maintaining the provider's inventory levels. The VMI reduces data entry errors, improves service levels (almost no stock-outs), and provides a platform for partnership working between providers and suppliers.[9] Information quality and management commitment are key to sustaining VMI in the long term. Healthcare managers should therefore consider committing to a vending relationship only after determining that it is possible to align both organisations in terms of information flow and quality.[65]

Collaborative planning and forecasting replenishment (CPFR) is another logistics tool that has received limited attention in healthcare. CPFR, originally defined by the Voluntary Interindustry Commerce Standards (VICS) Association,[66] is a collaborative technique that formalises the process of supply chain members

jointly agreeing a business plan and forecast, monitoring replenishment, and identifying and responding to any issues. The main purpose is to avoid a fragmented and
inefficient forecasting 'push' system, where companies predict customer demand
and products are 'pushed' through the supply chain (e.g. via distributors/
retailers) in anticipation of customer purchases. When replaced by a well-
coordinated and demand-driven 'pull' system that rapidly responds to the
requirements of the customer, there is less chance of stock-outs, and service
levels can be improved.

4.2.1 Inventory Management

Inappropriate inventory management can result in substantial losses for healthcare organisations and negatively impact on the quality and safety of patient
care.[67] Several reviews have examined how material flows are managed in
healthcare supply chains, including key areas such as logistics, procurement,
demand, and inventory management.[6,10,63,68,69] These have identified, for
example, that just-in-time (JIT) attempts to precisely match the demand for
care with goods/services, enabling suppliers and providers to deliver in small
quantities as and when required. Minimum stock levels and replenishment times
are calculated to avoid stock-outs and obsolete stock. They also require close
relations to be developed between healthcare organisations and suppliers.
Further, while maintaining the right inventory is a challenge for any healthcare
organisation, few hospital information systems can adequately capture data
relating to patient demand, process, or supplier performance.

Much attention has been given to the optimisation of inventory management
of pharmaceutical products. As noted earlier, these supply chains are continually challenged to manage the uncertainty of demand for pharmaceutical products and to reduce or remove the risk of product shortages, inventory that is no
longer needed, and counterfeits. In the era of artificial intelligence and the
introduction of more sophisticated inventory management systems, it is likely
that a shift to systems to mitigate the challenges and provide more flexible
solutions to resemble real-world situations will occur.[70]

4.2.2 Improving Flow of Materials and Supplies

Another approach used to improve the flow of materials involves classifying
materials by volume and frequency – known as runners, repeaters, and strangers –
to help coordinate and stream activities.[71] 'Runners' are products or services that
may be produced or delivered on a daily basis (e.g. ward rounds, observations)
and have enough demand to justify dedicated resources. 'Repeaters' are products
or services with intermediate but sufficient demand to warrant dedicated

resources. The quantity of repeaters may vary, but timings remain constant (e.g. weekly clinics), offering advantages in terms of ordering from suppliers, scheduling maintenance, and the availability of resources and equipment. A 'stranger' product or service has low or intermittent volume; the making of these products (or delivery of these services) must be fitted around the production slots of regular repeaters (see Bicheno and Holweg[72] for a detailed discussion).

Achieving the benefits of this approach may not be straightforward if patterns of demand for provision are not known or if patients' resource needs are not recognised across the different processes or pathways.[73,74] This can have consequences for the design of the healthcare supply chain or patient journey. To ensure a seamless transition from one healthcare provider to the next and from one operational approach to another, organisations need to consider how to coordinate care and communicate across organisational boundaries.

4.3 Supply Chain Design and Process Improvement

The supply chain (and improvement) literature often distinguishes between two major design/improvement paradigms – Lean and Agile. Lean can be described as 'containing little fat', potentially relating to the entire supply chain (from raw materials to the end consumer). Boundaries between organisations are seen as artificial, and value, as defined by the customer, is to be created at all stages of the supply chain.[75] Agile is characterised as 'nimble',[76] defined as 'a business wide capability that embraces organisational structures, information systems, logistics processes and, in particular, mindsets. A key characteristic of an Agile organisation or supply chain is flexibility.[77] Both Lean and Agile have been widely used in industry as mechanisms for designing and improving the performance of supply chains. In healthcare, Lean has received most attention, mainly in areas of process improvement rather than supply chain design.

4.3.1 Lean Supply Chains

Features of a Lean supply chain are:

- open and good levels of communication and information sharing
- strict quality processes and measurement systems
- limited number of suppliers
- long-term collaborations based on mutual trust
- early involvement of supply chain members in design/improvement activity
- effective feedback loops, sharing of risks and benefits, and working together to establish the best outcome for all parties.[78]

The car manufacturer Toyota is well known for removing waste and non-value adding activity from all tiers of its supply chain, which enabled the company to improve performance on delivery times, quality, and cost. The company first improved its internal functioning and then worked with its direct (first-tier) suppliers, who were strategic to its business, to improve their performance. By building long-term, collaborative relationships with suppliers, Toyota was able to focus both their own and suppliers' efforts on improving performance. It was then the responsibility of first-tier suppliers to cascade their learning to second-tier suppliers, and so on. This kind of approach can improve transparency within the supply chain, reduce the levels of inventory, and improve the quality and delivery of components. Trust and good communication are critical.[79,80]

A scoping review of the implementation of Lean in healthcare supply chains identified a significant increase in publications since 2013.[80] Most studies (30/54 papers) evaluated the activities of internal supply chains, with only three papers focusing on the processes of external supply chains. Examples of internal supply chains within one organisation included:

- preoperative[81]
- radiology[82]
- maternity[83]
- sterilisation[84]
- pharmaceutical.[85,86,87,88]

Examples of external supply chains included supply from a newly formed sterilisation service centre[89] and operations of a laundry service to reduce energy consumption.[90] The most prominent area of Lean practice was process mapping, which was used to gain an understanding of flow (e.g. materials, patients), eliminate waste (non-value adding activities), and identify improvement opportunities in the supply chain (e.g. introduction of JIT). Many of the studies failed to provide sufficient detail about the supply chains studied and the extent to which Lean was used to improve the design and performance.

4.3.2 Agile Supply Chains

Agile was introduced to manufacturing in response to the levels of uncertainty and change that organisations were facing.[91] Towill and Christopher define the characteristics of an Agile healthcare system as:

- a co-produced, patient-centred, or person-centred approach to commissioning
- the ability to deliver care to patient demand and expectation
- a holistic approach to service design that integrates healthcare providers, business processes, commissioners, and patients

- organisations having the ability to create new productive capability from the expertise of people and physical facilities regardless of their internal and external location.[76]

Perhaps surprisingly given the level of responsiveness, flexibility, adaptability, and speed required within most areas of healthcare, Agile as a strategy to improve healthcare supply chains has received less attention than Lean in the published literature.[92] Some supply chain scholars did support Agile supply chains as better placed to respond to the supply chain disruptions during the COVID-19 pandemic,[93] since responsiveness, information sharing, integration and data accessibility, cooperation, and flexibility were critical – especially for fast-moving goods such as personal protective equipment (PPE) and pharmaceuticals.

More recently, the concept of Agile healthcare has been linked with co-production and person-centred care.[27] As with other supply chain approaches, this positioning responds to the need for a highly responsive and flexible service to deliver good-quality healthcare to patients as and when they need it. Agility is also seen as valuable for humanitarian supply chains because it enables an efficient, resilient, and well-coordinated response to disaster (see Section 3.4). A benefit here is that an Agile system places emphasis on in-country capacity and a variety of agencies and providers coordinated within low-income countries or the 'global south', rather than being led by high-income countries.

4.3.3 Leagile Supply Chains

Much debate concerns whether Lean or Agile is most suited to managing supply chains. Some advocate that in a stable environment of high volume and low variation, Lean should be the choice. But in a more volatile environment that requires greater flexibility, an Agile supply chain might be recommended. The work of Naylor et al.[94] made a case for a hybrid approach combining both Lean and Agile – Leagility – that attempts to capitalise on the benefits of both.

The 'Leagile' hybrid approach to supply chain design proposes that Lean is most suited to upstream activities, which are mainly based on forecasts, and that Agile is best for downstream activities where demand is known and visible.[94] A Leagile approach is possible if it is clear where the movement (known as the decoupling point) from one approach to the other occurs (see Guven-Uslu et al.[95]).

As noted earlier, possibly the most well-known industry case for a hybrid approach is Zara, the Spanish fast-fashion clothing company. Zara is credited with developing one of the most effective quick-response systems in the garment industry. Its internal activities are designed to cope with high volumes and cost-efficiency of dying, cutting, labelling, and packaging. Other more specialised and labour-intensive finishing activities are outsourced to a network of small subcontractors who work on specific elements of the manufacturing process or types of garments. Some fabrics are also held un-dyed and unprinted to enable the company to respond quickly should demand be higher than expected. This hybrid approach shows that Lean can be used to reduce variation, standardise, and remove non-value activities. Specialist skills can then be applied to areas of the supply chain that need to be more adaptive and flexible, so require more Agile approaches.

In healthcare, while there are few studies to date, it has been suggested that upstream activities (Lean) could support public health interventions associated with long-term, preventative care, while downstream, more short-term activities relating to the treatment of disease might be more suited to Agile.[96] However, healthcare supply chains (such as care pathways) do appear to be suited to combinations of Lean and Agile, perhaps using the point of diagnosis as a decoupling point, with the level of criticality determining the sequence of and allocation of skills, expertise, and resources. A study conducted by Rahimnia and Moghadasian[97] considers how the decoupling point concept can be applied in three areas of a healthcare delivery system. They examine the decoupling of patient services in three identified treatment flows – rupture, fracture, and serious injuries – in a specialised hospital that treats trauma and injury. The decoupling point for this supply chain was located at the point of diagnosis of the injury, which distinguished between the three flows. Locating the decoupling point at this stage enables healthcare professionals to identify which patients require a more Agile and quick response.

A review of the humanitarian supply chain literature focused on pre-disaster and post-disaster phases found that both Lean and Agile support a rapid response at scale with the minimum of cost. The agility of the supply chain design is particularly beneficial in the response phase where a fast and customised approach is needed to provide the right aid in the right place.[98]

4.3.4 Decoupling of Front Office and Back Office

Another form of decoupling focuses on front-office and back-office activities. This is where activities are separated according to whether they are customer facing (front office) or not (back office). Back-office processes can be designed for efficiency using Lean (e.g. diagnostics in laboratories). One way to improve efficiency further is to move more front-office activity to the back office.[99] In healthcare, a front-office activity would involve some interaction with a patient or relative (e.g. pre-assessment before surgery, admission at outpatient clinic), while a back-office activity would be void of any interaction (e.g. testing of blood samples).[27] Front-office activity might require staff to be responsive (Agile) to the requirements of the patient.

Williams[27] examined the design of a respiratory pathway for patients with chronic obstructive pulmonary disease, distinguishing between back-office and front-office activities. Referrals from GPs to consultant or assessment clinics were back-office activities, whereas consultations, assessments, and pulmonary rehabilitation were front-office activities, since they require the patient's involvement. Usually, back-office activity is where Lean improvements can be made. Referrals were being made in several ways and with variable information, often leading to delay. In this case, standardising the referral process to a pulmonary rehabilitation programme could ensure that the rehabilitation team is provided with all vital information by every referrer, making the process of assessment and acceptance onto the programme more efficient. Making improvements to the back-office activity could save time that could then be spent on front-office activity with the patient (assuming the same resources were involved in back-office and front-office activity).

When considering decoupling activities, it is important to note that front-office work can vary in terms of the levels of interaction, customisation,[100] and contact time,[101] as well as the level of contact and degree of complexity of the transaction. All these points need to be considered carefully prior to dividing any activities, particularly in healthcare as it increasingly offers greater involvement of patients in how their care is delivered. Focusing on standardising back-office activities, often in the interest of efficiency and minimising costs, could also limit customisation (patient-centredness) and employee discretion.[101]

4.4 Managing and Improving Patient Flows

Notably, much supply chain and logistics research has focused on the flow of materials, supplies, and equipment. Yet understanding and managing patient flows (see the Element on Lean and other techniques for process improvement)[102] has been a longstanding and costly challenge for healthcare organisations as they strive to smooth the flow of elective surgery, reduce waits for inpatient admissions through emergency departments, achieve timely and efficient transfer of patients from intensive care units to medical or surgical wards, reduce patients' length of stay, and improve flow from inpatient care to long-term care facilities.[101,102] Patient logistics often concentrate on decisions regarding the variability and complexity of demand within a hospital, but important coordination issues also arise between different health and social care providers. Many optimisation questions in healthcare relate to the problem of matching high use of resources with high customer service levels.

Simulation and modelling can play an important role in understanding patient flows and managing demand and capacity. Accurate and reliable models of patient flow enable hospital managers to predict future activity. Such predictions are useful in assessing future bed usage and demands on various hospital resources, such as the number of beds required, and the associated staffing levels needed. From an operational perspective, patient flow represents the movement of patients through a set of locations in a healthcare facility.[103] Operational models of patient flow are very detailed and complex, usually taking the form of simulated queuing systems (for an example, see Bae et al.[104]). Although capable of providing very accurate predictions for various future system activities, these models can be costly and time-consuming to build and cannot be easily generalised. The expertise to develop such models may not be readily available to healthcare organisations.

In hospital settings, patient flow modelling has been applied to various scenarios (see Bhattacharjee and Ray[105]) but modelling of patient flows in other settings has remained less common. Palmer et al.'s[106] systematic review, focusing on the modelling of patient flows within community healthcare services, reports that few models consider the interaction between different services and the different mix of patients and how comorbidities are managed. This level of complexity suggests that a more agile approach is needed – one that responds quickly to the individual needs of those patients being cared for in the community.

Similarly, Ziat et al.[107] advocate for a distinctive approach to healthcare SCM. They argue that the fundamental purpose of the healthcare supply chain is to guarantee the quality and safety of patient care in a very complex and often resource-constrained environment. Using a framework to simultaneously describe both patient and material flow in a hospital environment helps to identify bottlenecks within the healthcare supply chain. Both flows rely on a well-coordinated information system to enable care to be delivered in a safe and timely manner. Identifying the processes within the patient and material flows supports good coordination and sequencing between the two flows to ensure that products and equipment are available as and when required but also helps prevent overstocking and wastage.

4.5 Advancing the Use of Digital Technologies and Data Analytics as a Way of Improving Supply Chains

Greater connectivity and standardisation across the supply chain has been enhanced by innovations such as barcodes and QR codes. A combination of technologies enhancing the connectivity and monitoring of supply chain members may help combat counterfeit medicines, product shortages, expiration, and recalls,[108] as well as increasing performance in terms of throughput[36] and limiting variability within the supply chain.

Technologies such as cloud-based and blockchain-based technology, the internet of things (connecting any device to the internet), chain of things (integrating the internet of things with blockchain networks), and artificial intelligence (simulating human intelligence in machines) have begun to revolutionise supply chains by seamlessly integrating providers and suppliers and improving quality and efficiency in the supply chain process.[108,109]

Blockchain technologies (also referred to as distributed ledgers because no one organisation or person controls the information) provide users with a unique, effective, and inexpensive way of exchanging currencies, maintaining accurate data, and facilitating contracts. These technologies, which include the use of smart sensors for real-time and predictive data analysis, can also support quick, safe, and secure solutions for tracking product authenticity from the start of production to the point of use.[108] Blockchain technologies have been used to provide a framework for product traceability and trusted information-sharing among supply chain stakeholders, with high integrity, security, and trust, and without the need for centralised intermediary governance or management.[117]

The move to more cloud-based platforms (i.e. the use of remote servers to handle data) has enhanced the opportunity to manage data on the high volume of products and materials used in any healthcare system. These platforms also offer the opportunity for live data-sharing to improve the traceability and security of the supply chain and establish direct access to patients and enable them to share information.[109] Cloud-based computer technologies can be used to bring together data from key supply chain members to generate accurate forecasts and production plans, as well as to automatically manage inventories and optimise transport routes.

The pharmaceutical supply chain is a good example of where 'edge devices' have been used to implement advanced solutions to improve transparency. Such devices collect data from sensors such as QR codes, radio frequency identification (RFID) tags, barcode readers, weighing scales, temperature sensors, GPS trackers, and supply chain visibility dashboards, which help to automate data collection, processing, and validation. They can ensure end-to-end coverage of the product lifecycle and improve visibility, traceability, and security across the supply chain.[110,111]

Big data analytics are also transforming supply chains by providing new insights into how organisations are performing based on data and statistical methods. Extensive use of data, statistical, and quantitative analysis, and explanatory and predictive modelling may encourage open and transparent decision-making and enable the simulation and optimisation of flows within the supply chain. Big data analytics are also important to enhance information-processing capacity and supply chain resilience for faster recovery after any disruptions.[112] Although digital technologies do enable large amounts of data to be collected on supply chains, the sharing of sensitive information, including patient data, is subject to tight regulation and governance. Various systems have been proposed to address data-sharing challenges, including those using new technologies (see, for example, Yue et al.[113] and Xia et al.[114]).

Advancements in technology are also likely to be important in supporting and limiting the environmental impact of healthcare supply chains. Sustainability and reverse flows (logistics) have become increasingly prominent in improving the management of the end-of-use and end-of-life of products and equipment. Both are often discussed within the wider context of the healthcare 'circular economy' where sustainable supply chains are prioritised, the use of healthcare products and equipment are prolonged, waste is minimised, and hazardous emissions are reduced or removed. A review by Campos et al.[115] of reverse logistics practices (recycling, reusing, and reducing) in the pharmaceutical industry found that operations practices, such as product recall, waste management, effluent treatment, reuse, recycling, donation, and incineration were all in use.

The key benefits of such technologies for healthcare supply chains are extended visibility and traceability, supply chain digitalisation, and improved data security.[116] Supply chain systems that embrace these technologies can share information in real time and allow organisations to make flexible adjustments according to changes in demand or supply.[117–119] Meanwhile, more intelligent processes and devices can effectively overcome the disadvantages of having different information systems in the supply chain, can maximise efficiency, and can create an intelligent, networked, and automated supply chain system.[120]

Despite the many potential benefits of these technologies, examples within healthcare supply chains tend to be limited to those associated more with the manufacture and movement of products such as medicines and vaccines. There are some instances where RFID has been used to track patients in hospitals in areas such as emergency departments, operating theatres, wards, and radiology,[121] but these studies are mainly focused on patient safety and generally not considered within the context of the wider supply chain.

4.6 Supply Chain Culture and Expertise

Notwithstanding some notable exceptions, culture and practices relating to supply chain and logistics are rarely central to the strategic vision of healthcare organisations.[122] Organisations often lack specialist supply chain skills, and logistics decisions are typically limited to the operational level rather than linked to strategic priorities. The reporting of shortages of critical items such as PPE and ventilators during the early stages of the COVID-19 pandemic was a critical moment for recognition of the importance of supply chains.[123] Until this time supply chain practitioners were often confused with procurement rather than a strategic role of managing national and often global supply chains. The pandemic made clear that healthcare needs to have well-designed supply chains that are resilient, responsive, and innovative when faced with threats.

Betcheva et al.[51] identify five operational challenges that need to be considered by healthcare and supply chain managers when developing and implementing a supply chain strategy.

1. **Greater coordination and integration** across the various supply chain members is needed to improve joint working and information sharing. In practice this can be challenging due to policies often focusing on the performance and payment to single organisations rather than encouraging joined-up working and integrated care.

2. **Standardisation** can relate to products, processes, tasks, and services and it is usually implemented to reduce or remove variability. Standardising the procurement of supplies and equipment can reduce costs through economies of scale and volume discounts. The standardisation of processes, using narrowly scoped tasks and standard operating procedures can enhance efficiency.

3. **Efficiency versus responsiveness**: Efficiencies can often be achieved using Lean principles and standardisation. High volume and low variation are key characteristics of these supply chains. Speciality providers such as the Shouldice Hospital in Canada, specialising in inguinal hernias, and Aravind Eye Hospitals in India, specialising in cataracts, are often quoted as examples of this approach.[51] In contrast, responsiveness is associated with flexible and agile practices (see Section 4.3) required to deal with unpredictable demand. As noted earlier, some healthcare supply chains may combine Lean and Agile to take the hybrid approach of Leagility to accommodate the different needs of the healthcare system.

4. **Pooling versus focused operations**: Pooling occurs through the redesign of supply activities and can result in cost savings and improved performance. For example, in healthcare pooling of procurement activity may happen where multiple hospitals route their spending through a group purchasing organisation, with the higher volumes resulting in lower prices. Pooling is not always the best option – a focused operation may be more effective. A study examining an Emergency Department pooled queuing system showed that the average waiting time and length of stay are longer when physicians are assigned patients under a pooled system when compared with a dedicated (similar) queuing system.[124]

5. **Incentive mechanisms,** whether financial or not, are employed to ensure all stakeholders are aligned to inter and intra-organisational goals within the supply chain. Incentivising information sharing – for example, the timeliness and accuracy of discharge summaries – can assist primary care physicians with the ongoing care of patients.[51] However, incentives can influence behaviour change, which may not always be aligned to the desired outcomes.

Empirical studies are required to enable us to understand how these challenges are addressed. As we indicate here, it may not be the case of selecting one approach but a combined or hybrid approach could be needed to deal with the complexities present in healthcare supply chains. Therefore it is imperative that supply chain skills and expertise continue to be supported and developed. Also critical will be ensuring that supply chain expertise works collaboratively with clinicians. For example, transfer of patients both within and between hospitals requires efficient logistics between internal and external supply chain partners (e.g. hospital, laboratory, and blood transfusion centre) as transfers generate significant costs and there is a potential danger of information loss or medical complication.[122] Supply chain professionals can play an important role in meeting clinicians' needs for evidence as care is redesigned.[123]

5 Critiques of the Supply Chain Management Improvement Approach

Healthcare needs to be well placed to provide patients and staff with the appropriate products and services, at the best price, in the right location, at the right time and right condition to achieve the best possible outcomes.[123] Managing supply chains is complex whatever the industry or service, and healthcare is no different. Challenges such as variability, inflexibility, and waste are frequently observed and difficult to manage,[124] with, for example, issues such as stock-outs and obsolete stock frequently occurring. The COVID-19 pandemic, with its shortages of key supplies at critical times, highlighted the need to manage and design supply chains differently not only in crisis situations but also to improve the responsiveness, resilience, and sustainability of healthcare supply chains more generally.[125,126]

Supply chain management has much to contribute to the improvement agenda in healthcare, but its potential has not yet been fully optimised, and the evidence base slow to build. Research designs other than questionnaire, simulation, and case-based research are limited. Experimental designs (including trials) and robust evaluation studies are very rare, particularly in the areas of supply chain design, performance, and improvement. There is little empirical evidence that measures the impact of SCM on the performance of healthcare services or patient pathways. Application of frameworks that have been used in other sectors such as the BSC and the SCOR models tend to be limited to a local level (e.g. internal supply chain) and within an acute care setting.[127,128] Where they have been extended to different healthcare settings, such as community and primary care, the adaptions made to the original framework to suit a specific healthcare context or supply chain are often unclear.[129] Notably, patients/families are rarely involved in the development of these frameworks, despite the ongoing drive for person-centred healthcare systems,[127] and the drive for person-centred care is not well reflected within the healthcare supply chain literature.[129] More guidance on how to robustly evaluate and report on the design and performance of healthcare supply chains is needed, and would enable areas of supply chain optimisation and good practice to be shared more widely within the sector.

Much of the available literature in healthcare has focused on internal supply chains. To some extent, this may reflect the maturity of SCM practice within healthcare, where organisations are looking to improve their internal supply chain processes before committing to larger, external improvements. There is less research focusing on end-to-end supply chains, despite the movement towards integrated health and social care services. There are very few examples which have widened the scope of the supply chain to include community and primary care.[27,127] This inward-looking and often limited view of the supply chain is similar to early research in manufacturing, which was restricted to one organisation.

Similarly, more 'manufacturing type' and 'product/equipment-based' supply chains (e.g. pharmaceutical, blood) tend to dominate the supply chain literature in healthcare, with Lean notably more prominent than Agility and Leagility. Research that robustly assesses these approaches is lacking. The ongoing debate around standardisation versus customisation (or person-centred care) has also not been fully addressed, while studies on information and financial flows, as well as workforce, have remained under-developed. These are important problems given the value of considering how product flows interact with other important flows, such as patients. Further exploration of how such flows can be modelled/mapped across the entire supply chain would help to visualise areas of good practice and identify where improvements need to be made. For example, giving more attention to workforce flows would help to assess utilisation of skills/expertise as well as identifying opportunities for inter-professional working.

What is clear from the available evidence is that collaboration, information-sharing, and coordination across organisational boundaries are prerequisites for sustainable, long-term relationships among key supply chain stakeholders. Yet how healthcare organisations work with their key suppliers and providers is not fully understood. We often see supplier development programmes in other sectors, but it is not clear what formal programmes are used to support joint product development and service/supply chain redesign in healthcare.

Advanced technologies (e.g. blockchain, RFID) in the design and operation of supply chains are poised to make a positive contribution to responsiveness, flexibility, and product security (e.g. reducing falsified and counterfeit medicines) and potentially an environmentally friendly circular economy. However, the challenges of ensuring the connectivity and governance arrangements to support the cross-organisation working and the visibility to support end-to-end supply chain activities need to be addressed. Holistic model testing that combines the impact of these technologies on the healthcare systems and supply chains is lacking. Further research is needed to fully assess the impact and possible trade-offs when investing in various digital technologies.[130]

6 Conclusions

In this Element, we have identified the strategic importance of SCM in healthcare but have also highlighted some of the key challenges and problems. The complexity of managing various flows of materials, equipment, patients, and finances across a network of suppliers and providers is evident. We have identified some of the strategies that can be used in SCM, such as improving efficiency, increasing responsiveness, better use of technology, and improving the processes and systems. We have identified that representation at a senior management level is critical to ensure that supply chain activity is continually aligned to the strategic vision of any healthcare organisation, and that supply chain skills and expertise (including procurement and logistics) need to be continually developed.

Supply chain management efforts in healthcare to date are often limited to internal supply chains and/or those associated with the manufacture of products, and research in the field has been similarly limited. As methods of SCM continue to emerge, they need to be studied, analysed, and evaluated for their performance and efficacy for use in general and in healthcare supply chain systems in particular.[131] Developing and advancing the evidence base will help us to better understand the nuances and complexities of SCM in healthcare. In Box 4, we set out several areas for further research that will contribute to our understanding and appreciation of SCM in healthcare.

The fundamental purpose of the healthcare supply chain is to support the quality and safety of patient care in a complex and often resource-constrained environment.[107] We have highlighted some of the areas where further developments can be made to advance the application of SCM within healthcare. Such advancements will contribute to the development and introduction of new models of care and the pursuit to continually improve patient outcomes.

Box 4 Areas for further research on SCM in healthcare

- **Supply chain strategy:** Greater insight to strategic positioning of SCM within and across healthcare systems is needed to provide clarity on the practical requirements in relation to design, governance, measurement, and impact. A critical assessment of structures, roles, and responsibilities to support the implementation of supply chain strategies is also required.

- **Understanding and managing flows:** As discussions move from a linear supply chain perspective to networks of organisations, each with their different (and misaligned) processes, systems, professional perspectives, and policies,[132] understanding and managing flows will become a particularly important area for future research. Most existing studies examine the movement of material, supplies, equipment, and, to some extent, patient flows; there are clear benefits to extending this to cover information and financial flows.

- **Integrated care networks:** Further research is required at a whole-systems level to provide a better understanding of healthcare supply chain networks that span integrated care networks, which might also include charities and third sector organisations. Supply chain management is well-placed to contribute to the design and delivery of new models of care.

- **What works and when:** Well-designed and executed studies (e.g. controlled trials or other experimental approaches) are required to enable further testing of supply chain practices and techniques. This will improve understanding of what works, for whom, and when, beyond more logistics-focused supply chains, which usually include product-related and information flows. Keeping pace with the advancements in the use of digital technologies and data analytics is fundamental to the design and development of resilient healthcare supply chains.

- **Testing of design concepts and supplier/provider development programmes:** Few healthcare organisations have invested in logistics and supply chain expertise despite their value for reducing variation and improving supply chain performance and resilience to enhance patient care. Design concepts such as decoupling (see Section 4.3.4), along with formal supplier/provider development programmes, have not yet been fully tested within a healthcare environment.

- **Environmental sustainability:** Further exploration is needed of the circular economy of healthcare to ensure that healthcare supply chain configurations are moving away from the 'take-make-consume-dispose' pattern of material flows to sustainable 'closed-loops' by combining processes 'such as maintenance, repair, reusing, refurbishing, remanufacturing, and recycling'.[133]

- **Workforce:** Further research is needed to contribute to a better understanding of the workforce supply chain, which will need to take a more collaborative approach to workforce planning across health and social care to identify and evaluate new roles and to constrain healthcare providers from having too strong a 'gravitational pull'[28] on social care.[24,28]

7 Further Reading

- Bicheno and Holweg[72] – this practical text provides details of many of the improvement tools and techniques now used in healthcare, including the concept of runners, repeaters, and strangers introduced in Section 3.1.
- Betcheva et al.[24] – provides an excellent insight into the design and operation of healthcare supply chains.
- Radnor et al.[136] – this edited book provides some useful case studies on healthcare operations management and supply chains.
- Schneller et al.[123] – the second edition of this key text considers the enablers and barriers to progressive supply chain management in healthcare.
- Williams[27] – this book provides two healthcare case studies to illustrate the concepts of Lean and Agile design in relation to two patient pathways.

Contributors

Conflicts of Interest

None.

Acknowledgements

The authors thank the peer reviewers and the THIS Institute team for their insightful comments and recommendations to improve the Element. A list of peer reviewers is published at www.cambridge.org/IQ-peer-reviewers.

Funding

This Element was funded by THIS Institute (The Healthcare Improvement Studies Institute, www.thisinstitute.cam.ac.uk). THIS Institute is strengthening the evidence base for improving the quality and safety of healthcare. THIS Institute is supported by a grant to the University of Cambridge from the Health Foundation – an independent charity committed to bringing about better health and healthcare for people in the United Kingdom.

About the Author

Sharon J. Williams is Professor of Healthcare Operations Management at Swansea University. Her background is in service operations and supply chain management and her interdisciplinary research aims to improve the quality of health and social care services by drawing on approaches used in other sectors.

Creative Commons License

References

1. Braithwaite J, Iedema RA, Jorm C. Trust, communication, theory of mind and social brain hypothesis: Deep explanations for what goes wrong in health care. *J Health Organ Manage* 2007; 21: 353–67. https://doi.org/10.1108/14777 260710778899.

2. Lee SM, Lee DH, Schniederjans MJ. Supply chain innovation and organizational performance in the healthcare industry. *Int J Operations Prod Manage* 2011; 31: 1193–214. https://doi.org/10.1108/01443571111178493.

3. Green LV. OM Forum – the vital role of operations analysis in improving healthcare delivery. *Manuf Serv Operations Manage* 2012; 14: 488–94. https://doi.org/10.1287/msom.1120.0397.

4. Böhme T, Williams SJ, Childerhouse P, Deakins E, Towill D. Methodology challenges associated with benchmarking healthcare supply chains. *Prod Plann Control* 2013; 24: 1002–14. https://doi.org/10.1080/09537287.2012.666918.

5. Böhme T, Williams S, Childerhouse P, Deakins E, Towill D. Squaring the circle of healthcare supplies. *J Health Organ Manage* 2014; 28: 247–65. https://doi.org/10.1108/JHOM-01-2013-0014.

6. Mathur B, Gupta S, Meena ML, Dangayach GS. Healthcare supply chain management: Literature review and some issues. *J Adv Manage Res* 2018; 15: 265–87. https://doi.org/10.1108/JAMR-09-2017-0090.

7. Beier F. The management of the supply chain for hospital pharmacies: A focus on inventory management practices. *J Bus Logist* 1995; 16: 153.

8. Elmuti D, Khoury G, Omran O, Abou-Zaid AS. Challenges and opportunities of health care supply chain management in the United States. *Health Mark Q* 2013; 30: 128–43. https://doi.org/10.1080/07359683.2013.787885.

9. Kwon I-W, Kim S-H, Martin DG. Healthcare supply chain management; strategic areas for quality and financial improvement. *Technol Forecast Soc Change* 2016; 113: 422–28. https://doi.org/10.1016/j.techfore.2016.07.014.

10. de Vries J, Huijsman R. Supply chain management in health services: An overview. *Supply Chain Manage* 2011; 16: 159–65. https://doi.org/10.1108/13598541111127146.

11. McKone-Sweet KE, Hamilton P, Willis SB. The ailing healthcare supply chain: A prescription for change. *J Supply Chain Manage* 2005; 41: 4–17. https://doi.org/10.1111/j.1745-493X.2005.tb00180.x.

12. Miller FA, Young SB, Dobrow M, Shojania KG. Vulnerability of the medical product supply chain: The wake-up call of COVID-19. *BMJ Qual Saf* 2021; 30: 331–35. http://dx.doi.org/10.1136/bmjqs-2020-012133.

13. Ranney ML, Griffeth V, Jha AK. Critical supply shortages – the need for ventilators and personal protective equipment during the Covid-19 pandemic. *N Engl J Med* 2020; 382: e41. https://doi.org/10.1056/NEJMp2006141.

14. Leite H, Lindsay C, Kumar M. COVID-19 outbreak: Implications on health-care operations. *TQM Journal* 2020; 33: 247–56. https://doi.org/10.1108/TQM-05-2020-0111.

15. Kelle P, Transchel S, Minner S. Buyer-supplier cooperation and negotiation support with random yield consideration. *Int J Product Econ* 2009; 118: 152–59. https://doi.org/10.1016/j.ijpe.2008.08.018.

16. Du Toit D, Vlok P-J. Supply chain management: A framework of understanding. *S Afr J Ind Eng* 2014; 25: 25–38. https://doi.org/10.7166/25-3-743.

17. Kritchanchai D, Krichanchai S, Hoeur S, Tan A. Healthcare supply chain management: Macro and micro perspectives. *LogForum* 2019; 15: 531–44. http://doi.org/10.17270/J.LOG.2019.371.

18. Ketchen DJ, Giunipero LC. The intersection of strategic management and supply chain management. *Ind Mark Manage* 2004; 33: 51–56. https://doi.org/10.1016/j.indmarman.2003.08.010.

19. Christopher M. Logistics and supply chain management, 5th ed. Harlow, England: Pearson Education; 2016.

20. Christopher M. Logistics and supply chain management, 2nd ed. London: Pitman; 1998.

21. Jindal RP, Gauri DK, Li W, Ma Y. Omnichannel battle between Amazon and Walmart: Is the focus on delivery the best strategy? *J Bus Res* 2021, 122: 270–80. https://doi.org/10.1016/j.jbusres.2020.08.053.

22. Aftab MA, Yuanjian Q, Kabir N, Barua Z. Super responsive supply chain: The case of Spanish fast fashion retailer Inditex-Zara. *Int J Bus Manage* 2018; 13: 212–27. https://doi.org/10.5539/ijbm.v13n5p212.

23. Meijboom B, Schmidt-Bakx S, Westert G. Supply chain management practices for improving patient-oriented care. *Supply Chain Manage* 2011; 16: 166–75. https://doi.org/10.1108/13598541111127155.

24. Betcheva L, Erhun F, Jiang H. Healthcare supply chains. In: Choi TY, Li JJ, Rogers DS, Schoenherr T, Wagner SM, editors. The Oxford handbook of supply chain management. New York: Oxford University Press; 2020.

25. Kelle P, Woosley J, Schneider H. Pharmaceutical supply chain specifics and inventory solutions for a hospital case. *Operations Res Health Care* 2012; 1: 54–63. https://doi.org/10.1016/j.orhc.2012.07.001.

26. Trebble TM, Hansi N, Hydes T, Smith MA, Baker M. Process mapping the patient journey: An introduction. *BMJ* 2010; 341: c4078. https://doi.org/10.1136/bmj.c4078.

27. Williams S. Improving healthcare operations: The application of Lean, Agile and Leagility in care pathway design. Cham, Switzerland: Palgrave Macmillan; 2017.

28. Beech J, Bottery S, Charlesworth A, et al. Closing the gap: Key areas for action on the health and care workforce. London: The Health Foundation, The King's Fund, Nuffield Trust; 2019. www.kingsfund.org.uk/publica tions/closing-gap-health-care-workforce (accessed 16 August 2021).

29. Warren, S. The health and care workforce: Planning for a sustainable future. London: The King's Fund; 2022. www.kingsfund.org.uk/publica tions/health-and-care-workforce#service-improvement-ambitions (accessed 10 August 2023).

30. Street A, Gutacker N. Health economics. In: Dixon-Woods M, Brown K, Marjanovic S, et al., editors. *Elements of Improving Quality and Safety in Healthcare*. Cambridge: Cambridge University Press; 2023. https://doi .org/10.1017/9781009325974.

31. Singh RK, Kumar R, Kumar P. Strategic issues in pharmaceutical supply chains: A review. *Int J Pharm Healthc Mark* 2016; 10: 234–57. https://doi .org/10.1108/IJPHM-10-2015-0050.

32. Papalexi M, Breen L, Bamford D, Tipi NS. (2014). A preliminary examination of the deployment of Lean and reverse logistics within the pharmaceutical supply chain (PSC) UK. In: LRN Annual Conference and PhD Workshop 3-5th Sept., University of Huddersfield (unpublished): 1–9. http://eprints.edu.ac.uk/eprint23230/.

33. Narayana SA, Pati RK, Vrat P. Managerial research on the pharmaceutical supply – a critical review and some insights for future directions. *J Purch Supply Manage* 2014; 20: 18–40. https://doi.org/10.1016/j.pursup.2013.09.001.

34. Halabi SF, Gostin L. Falsified and substandard medicines in globalized pharmaceutical supply chains: Toward actionable solutions. In: Halabi SF, editor. Food and drug regulation in an era of globalized markets. 2015: 51–61. San Diego, CA: Academic Press.

35. Chung SH, Kwon C. Integrated supply chain management for perishable products: Dynamics and oligopolistic competition perspectives with application to pharmaceuticals. *Int J Product Econ* 2016; 179: 117–29. https:// doi.org/10.1016/j.ijpe.2016.05.021.

36. Jamil F, Hang L, Kim K, Kim D. A novel medical blockchain model for drug supply chain integrity management in a smart hospital. *Electronics* 2019; 8: 505. https://doi.org/10.3390/electronics8050505.

37. Duijzer LE, van Jaarsveld W, Dekker R. Literature review: The vaccine supply chain. *Eur J Oper Res* 2018; 268: 174–92. https://doi.org/10.1016/j.ejor .2018.01.015.

38. World Health Organization. Covid-19 vaccination: Supply and logistics guidance. Interim guidance. Geneva: WHO. www.who.int/publications/i/item/who-2019-ncov-vaccine-deployment-logistics-2021-1 (accessed 25 May 2022).

39. Lemmens S, Decouttere C, Vandaele N, Bernuzzi M. A review of integrated supply chain network design models: Key issues for vaccine supply chains. *Chem Eng Res Des* 2016; 109: 366–84. https://doi.org/10.1016/j.cherd.2016.02.015.

40. Beliën J, Forcé H. Supply chain management of blood products: A literature review. *Eur J Oper Res* 2012; 217: 1–16. https://doi.org/10.1016/j.ejor.2011.05.026.

41. de Oliveira Mota D, Monteleone JP, Pessoa JLE, Pimentel CFMG. São Paulo state liver transplantation supply chain study. *Transplant Proc* 2020; 53: 1247–50. https://doi.org/10.1016/j.transproceed.2020.02.181.

42. Oloruntoba R, Gray R. Humanitarian aid: An Agile supply chain? *Supply Chain Manage* 2006; 11: 115–20. https://doi.org/10.1108/13598540610652492

43. Bhattacharya S, Hasija S, Van Wassenhove LN. Designing efficient infrastructural investment and asset transfer mechanisms in humanitarian supply chains. *Prod Operations Manage* 2014; 23: 1511–121. https://doi.org/10.1111/poms.12177.

44. Holguín-Veras J, Jaller M, Van Wassenhove LN, Pérez N, Wachtendorf T. On the unique features of post-disaster humanitarian logistics. *J Operations Manage* 2012; 30: 494–506. http://dx.doi.org/10.1016/j.jom.2012.08.003.

45. Dubey R, Altay N, Blome C. Swift trust and commitment: The missing links for humanitarian supply chain coordination? *Ann Operations Res* 2019; 283: 159–77. https://doi.org/10.1007/s10479-017-2676-z.

46. Duong LNK, Chong J. Supply chain collaboration in the presence of disruptions: A literature review. *Int J Product Res* 2020; 58: 3488–507. https://doi.org/10.1080/00207543.2020.1712491.

47. Kovács G, Spens KM. Humanitarian logistics in disaster relief operations. *Int J Phys Distrib Logist Manage* 2007; 37: 99–114. https://doi.org/10.1108/09600030710734820.

48. Kovács G, Spens KM. Trends and developments in humanitarian logistics – a gap analysis. *Int J Physical Distrib Logist Manage* 2011; 41: 32–45. https://doi.org/10.1108/09600031111101411.

49. Seifert L, Kunz N, Gold S. Humanitarian supply chain management responding to refugees: A literature review. *J Humanitarian Logist Supply Chain Manage* 2018; 8: 398–426. https://doi.org/10.1108/JHLSCM-07-2017-0029.

50. Jackson TL, editor. *5S for healthcare*. New York: Productivity Press; 2009.

51. Betcheva L, Erhun F, Jiang H. OM forum – supply chain thinking in healthcare: Lessons and outlooks. *Manuf Serv Operations Manage* 2020; 23: 1333–53. https://doi.org/10.1287/msom.2020.0920.

52. Kaplan R, Norton D. The balanced scorecard – measures that drive performance. *Harv Bus Rev* 1992; 70: 71–79. https://hbr.org/1992/01/the-balanced-scorecard-measures-that-drive-performance-2.

53. Stewart, G. Supply-chain operations reference model (SCOR): The first cross-industry framework for integrated supply chain management. *Logist Inf Manag* 1997; 10(2): 62–67. https://doi.org/10.1108/0957605971 0815716.

54. Lenin K. Measuring supply chain performance in the healthcare industry. *Sci J Bus Manage* 2014; 2: 136–42. https://doi.org/10.11648/j.sjbm .20140205.14.

55. Moons K, Waeyenbergh G, Pintelon L. Measuring the logistics performance of internal hospital supply chains – a literature study. *Omega* 2019; 82: 205–17. https://doi.org/10.1016/j.omega.2018.01.007.

56. Stevens GC, Johnson M. Integrating the supply chain … 25 years on. *Int J Phys Distrib Logist Manage* 2016; 46: 19–42. https://doi.org/ 10.1108/IJPDLM-07-2015-0175.

57. Schmenner RW, Swink ML. On theory in operations management. *J Operations Manage* 1998; 17: 97–113. https://doi.org/10.1016/S0272-6963(98)00028-X.

58. Towill DR. The seamless supply chain – the predator's strategic advantage. *Int J Technol Manage* 1997; 13: 37–56. https://doi.org/10.1504/IJTM.1997 .001649.

59. Senge PM. *The fifth discipline: The art and practice of the learning organization*. London: Random House; 1994.

60. Parnaby J, Towill DR. Seamless healthcare delivery systems. *Int J Health Care Qual Assur* 2008; 21: 249–73. https://doi.org/10.1108/095268608 10868201.

61. Fisher ES, Staiger DO, Bynum JPW, Gottlieb DJ. Creating accountable care organizations: The extended hospital medical staff. *Health Aff* 2006; 25: W44–W57. https://doi.org/10.1377/hlthaff.26.1.w44.

62. Coleman BJ, Jennings KM. The UPS strike: Lessons for just-in-timers. *Product Inventory Manage J* 1998; 39: 63–68.

63. Kim S-H, Kwon I-WG. The study of healthcare supply chain management in United States: Literature review. *Manage Rev Int J* 2015; 10: 34–56. www.researchgate.net/profile/Sung-Ho-Kim-3/publication/334223774_ The_Study_of_Healthcare_Supply_Chain_Management_in_United_States_

Literature_Review/links/5db56c24a6fdccc99da3fb3b/The-Study-of-Healthcare-Supply-Chain-Management-in-United-States-Literature-Review.pdf (accessed 30 April 2022).

64. Doone R. How supply chain management can help to control health-care costs. *Supply Chain Q* 2014; 3: 50–53. www.supplychainquarterly.com/articles/914-how-supply-chain-management-can-help-to-control-health-care-costs (accessed 25 May 2022).

65. Falasca M, Kros JF. Success factors and performance outcomes of healthcare industrial vending systems: An empirical analysis. *Technol Forecast Soc Change* 2018; 126: 41–52. https://doi.org/10.1016/j.techfore.2016.06.024.

66. Panahifar M, Heavey C, Byrne P, Fazlollahtabar H. A framework for collaborative planning, forecasting and replenishment (CPFR): State of the art. *J Enterp Inf Manag* 2015; 28(6): 838–71. https://doi.org/10.1108/JEIM-09-2014-0092.

67. Brandon-Jones E, Squire B, Autry C, Petersen K. A contingent resource-based perspective of supply chain resilience and robustness. *J Supply Chain Manag* 2014; 50(3): 55–73. https://doi.org/10.1111/jscm.12050.

68. Dixit A, Routroy S, Dubey SK. A systematic literature review of healthcare supply chain and implications of future research. *Int J Pharm Healthc Mark* 2019; 13: 405–35. https://doi.org/10.1108/IJPHM-05-2018-0028.

69. Leaven L, Ahmmad K, Peebles D. Inventory management applications for healthcare supply chains. *Int J Supply Chain Manage* 2017; 6: 1–7. http://ijis-scm.bsne.ch/ojs.excelingtech.co.uk/index.php/IJSCM/article/download/1601/1601-5978-1-PB.pdf (accessed 30 April 2022).

70. Ahmadi E, Mosadegh H, Maihami R et al. Intelligent inventory management approaches for perishable pharmaceutical products in a healthcare supply chain. *Comput Oper Res* 2022; 147. https://doi.org/10.1016/j.cor.2022.105968.

71. Walley P, Silvester K, Steyn R. Managing variation in demand: Lessons from the UK National Health Service. *J Healthc Manage* 2006: 51: 309–20.

72. Bicheno J, Holweg M. The Lean toolbox: The essential guide to Lean transformation, 4th ed. Buckingham: PICSIE Books; 2009.

73. Walley P. Does the public sector need a more demand-driven approach to capacity management? *Prod Plann Control* 2013; 24: 877–90. https://doi.org/10.1080/09537287.2012.666886.

74. Glenday I. Moving to flow (levelled production). *Manuf Eng* 2005; 84: 20–23. https://doi.org/10.1049/me:20050203.

75. Lamming R. Squaring Lean supply with supply chain management. *Int J Operations Prod Manage* 1996; 16: 183–96. https://doi.org/10.1108/01443579610109910.

76. Towill D, Christopher M. The supply chain strategy conundrum: To be Lean or Agile or to be Lean and Agile? *Int J Logist Res Appl* 2002; 3: 299–309. https://doi.org/10.1080/1367556021000026736.

77. Christopher M. The Agile supply chain: Competing in volatile markets. *Ind Mark Manage* 2000; 29: 37–44. https://doi.org/10.1016/S0019-8501(99)00110-8.

78. Martínez-Jurado J, Moyano-Fuentes J. Lean management, supply chain management and sustainability: A literature review. *J Cleaner Product* 2014; 85: 134–50. https://doi.org/10.1016/j.jclepro.2013.09.042.

79. Hines P. *Creating world-class suppliers: Unlocking mutual competitive advantage*. London: Pitman; 1994.

80. Borges GA, Tortorella G, Rossini M, Portioli-Staudacher A. Lean implementation in healthcare supply chain: A scoping review. *J Health Organ Manage* 2019; 33: 304–22. https://doi.org/10.1108/JHOM-06-2018-0176.

81. Kimsey D. Lean methodology in health care. *AORN J* 2010; 92(1): 53–60. https://doi.org/10.1016/j.aorn.2010.01.015.

82. Donnelly G, Forester L, Donnelly L. Reliable and efficient supply chain management in radiology: Implementation of a two-bin demand-flow system. *J Am Coll Radiol* 2016; 13(4): 426–28. https://doi.org/10.1016/j.jacr.2015.09.006.

83. Kumar S, Swanson E, Tran T. RFID in the healthcare supply chain: Usage and application. *Int JHealth Care Qual Assur* 2009; 22(1): 67–81. https://doi.org/10.1108/09526860910927961.

84. Kumar A, Rahman S. RFID-enabled process reengineering of closed-loop supply chains in the healthcare industry of Singapore. *J Clean Prod* 2014; 85: 382–94. https://doi.org/10.1016/j.jclepro.2014.04.037.

85. Jahre M, Dumoulin L, Greenhalgh L et al. Improving health in developing countries: Reducing complexity of drug supply chains. *J Humanit* 2012; 2(1): 54–84. https://doi.org/10.1108/20426741211226000.

86. Guimaraes CM, Crespo De Carvalho J, Maia A. Vendor Managed Inventory (VMI): Evidences from lean deployment in healthcare. *Strat Outsourc* 2013; 6(1): 8–24. https://doi.org/10.1108/17538291311316045.

87. Papalexi M, Bamford D, Dehe B. A case study of kanban implementation within the pharmaceutical supply chain. *Int J Logist Res Appl* 2016; 19(4): 239–255. https://doi.org/10.1080/13675567.2015.1075478.

88. Nabelsi V, Gagnon S. Information technology strategy for a patient-oriented, lean, and agile integration of hospital pharmacy and medical equipment supply chains. *Int J Prod Res* 2017; 55(14): 3929–45. https://doi.org/10.1080/00207543.2016.1218082.

89. Kumar A, Ozdamar L, Ning Zhang C. Supply chain redesign in the healthcare industry of Singapore. *Supply Chain Manag* 2008; 13(2): 95–103. https://doi.org/10.1108/13598540810860930.

90. Zhu Q, Johnson S, Sarkis J. Lean six sigma and environmental sustainability: A hospital perspective. *Supply Chain Forum* 2018; 19(1): 25–41. https://doi.org/10.1080/16258312.2018.1426339.

91. Ismail HS, Sharifi H. A balanced approach to building agile supply chains. *Int J Phys Distrib Logist Manage* 2006; 36: 431–44. https://doi.org/10.1108/09600030610677384.

92. Patri R, Suresh, M. Agility in healthcare services: A systematic literature exploration. *Int J Serv Oper Manag* 2019; 32(3): 387–404. https://doi.org/10.1504/IJSOM.2019.098356.

93. Tonday H, Katore P, Raut D, Rathod A, Morwal A. Study of implementation of agile supply chain for efficient delivery of essentials during Covid-19. *SSRG Int J Mech Eng* 2021; 8(8): 1–6. https://doi.org/10.14445/23488360/IJME-V8I8P101.

94. Naylor JB, Naim MN, Berry D. Leagility: Integrating the Lean and Agile manufacturing paradigms in the total supply chain. *Int J Product Econ* 1999; 62: 107–18. https://doi.org/10.1016/S0925-5273(98)00223-0.

95. Guven-Uslu P, Chan HK, Ijaz S, Bak O, Whitlow B, Kumar V. In-depth study of 'decoupling point' as a reference model: An application for health service supply chain. *Prod Plann Control* 2014; 25: 1107–17. https://doi.org/10.1080/09537287.2013.808841.

96. Marshall L, Finch D, Cairncross L, Bibby J. Briefing: The Nation's health as an asset: Building the evidence on the social and economic value of health. London: The Health Foundation; 2018. www.health.org.uk/publications/the-nations-health-as-an-asset.

97. Rahimnia F, Moghadasian M. Supply chain leagility in professional services: How to apply decoupling point concept in healthcare delivery system. *Supply Chain Manage* 2010; 15: 80–91. https://doi.org/10.1108/13598541011018148.

98. Upadhyay A, Mukhuty S, Kumari S, Garza-Reyes JA, Shukla V. A review of Lean and Agile management in humanitarian supply chains: Analysing the pre-disaster and post-disaster phases and future directions. *Prod Plann Control* 2020; 33: 641–54. https://doi.org/10.1080/09537287.2020.1834133.

99. Chase RB, Tansik DA. The customer contact model for organization design. *Manage Sci* 1983; 29: 1037–50. https://doi.org/10.1287/mnsc.29.9.1037.

100. Schmenner RW. How can service businesses survive and prosper? *Sloan Manage Rev* 1986; 27: 21–32.

101. Silvestro R, Fitzgerald L, Johnston R, Voss C. Towards a classification of service processes. *Int J Serv Ind Manage* 1992; 3: 62–75. https://doi.org/ 10.1108/09564239210015175.

102. Radnor Z, Williams S. Lean and associated techniques for process improvement. In: Dixon-Woods M, Brown K, Marjanovic S et al., editors. *Elements of Improving Quality and Safety in Healthcare*. Cambridge: Cambridge University Press; forthcoming.

103. Marshall A, Vasilakis C, El-Darzi E. Length of stay-based patient flow models: Recent developments and future directions. *Health Care Manage Sci* 2005; 8: 213–20. https://doi.org/10.1007/s10729-005-2012-z.

104. Bae K-H, Jones M, Evans G, Antimisiaris D. Simulation modelling of patient flow and capacity planning for regional long-term care needs: A case study. *J Health Syst* 2019; 8: 1–16. https://doi.org/10.1080/ 20476965.2017.1405873.

105. Bhattacharjee P, Ray PK. Patient flow modelling and performance analysis of healthcare delivery processes in hospitals: A review and reflections. *Comput Ind Eng* 2014; 78: 299–312. https://doi.org/10.1016/ j.cie.2014.04.016.

106. Palmer R, Fulop NJ, Utley M. A systematic literature review of operational research methods for modelling patient flow and outcomes within community healthcare and other settings. *Health Systems* 2018; 7: 29–50. https://doi.org/10.1057/s41306-017-0024-9.

107. Ziat A, Sefiani N, Reklaoui K, Azzouzi H. A generic framework for hospital supply chain. *Int J Healthc Manage* 2019; 13: 488–95. www .doi.org/10.1080/20479700.2019.1603415.

108. Sathiya V, Nagalakshmi K, Jeevamalar J et al. Reshaping healthcare supply chain using chain-of-things technology and key lessons experienced from Covid-19 pandemic. *Socio-Econ Plan Sci* 2023; 85: 101510. https://doi.org/10.1016/j.seps.2023.101510.

109. Lu Y. Artificial intelligence: A survey on evolution, models, applications and future trends. *J Manage Anal* 2019; 6: 1–29. https://doi.org/10.1080/ 23270012.2019.1570365.

110. Papert M, Rimpler P, Pflaum A. Enhancing supply chain visibility in a pharmaceutical supply chain: Solutions based on automatic identification technology. *Int J Phys Distrib Logist Manage* 2016; 46: 859–84. https://doi.org/10.1108/IJPDLM-06-2016-0151.

111. Botcha KM, Chakravarthy V, Anurag. Enhancing traceability in pharmaceutical supply chain using Internet of Things (IoT) and Blockchain. *IEEE Int Conf Intell Syst Green Technol (ICISGT)* 2019; 45–453. https://doi.org/ 10.1109/ICISGT44072.2019.00025.

112. Dubey R, Gunasekaran A, Childe SJ et al. Empirical investigation of data analytics capability and organizational flexibility as complements to supply chain resilience. *Int J Product Res* 2021; 59: 110–28. https://doi.org/10.1080/00207543.2019.1582820.

113. Yue X, Wang H, Jin D, Li M, Jiang W. Healthcare data gateways: Found healthcare intelligence on blockchain with novel privacy risk control. *J Med Syst* 2016; 40: 218. https://doi.org/10.1007/s10916-016-0574-6.

114. Xia Q, Sifah EB, Smahi A, Amofa S, Zhang X. BBDS: Blockchain-Based Data Sharing for electronic medical records in cloud environments. Information 2017; 8: 44. https://doi.org/10.3390/info8020044.

115. Campos EARd, Paula ICd, Pagani RN, Guarnieri P. Reverse logistics for the end-of-life and end-of-use products in the pharmaceutical industry: A systematic literature review. *Supply Chain Manage* 2017; 22: 375–92. https://doi.org/10.1108/SCM-01-2017-0040.

116. Wang Y, Han JH, Beynon-Davies P. Understanding blockchain technology for future supply chains: A systematic literature review and research agenda. *Supply Chain Manage* 2019; 24: 62–84. https://doi.org/10.1108/SCM-03-2018-0148.

117. Teixeira KC, Borsato M. Development of a model for the dynamic formation of supplier networks. *J Ind Inf Integration* 2019; 15: 161–73. https://doi.org/10.1016/j.jii.2018.11.007.

118. Zandieh M, Aslani B. A hybrid MCDM approach for order distribution in a multiple-supplier supply chain: A case study. *J Ind Inf Integration* 2019; 16: 100104. https://doi.org/10.1016/j.jii.2019.08.002.

119. Zhang R, Wang K. Service supply chain research: A conceptual model based on business processes. *J Ind Integration Manage* 2019; 4: 1950007. https://doi.org/10.1142/S2424862219500076.

120. Nabhani F, Uhl C, Kauf F, Shokri A. Supply chain process optimisation via the management of variance. *J Manage Anal* 2018; 5: 136–53. https://doi.org/10.1080/23270012.2018.1424571.

121. Ebrahimzadeh F, Nabovati E, Hasibian M, Esalmi S. Evaluation of the effects of radio-frequency identification technology on patient tracking in hospitals: A systematic review. *J Patient Saf* 2021; 17(8): e1157–65. https://doi.org/10.1097/PTS.0000000000000446.

122. Ageron B, Benzidia S, Bourlakis M. Healthcare logistics and supply chain – issues and future challenges. *Supply Chain Forum* 2018; 19: 1–3, https://doi.org/10.1080/16258312.2018.1433353.

123. Schneller, E. Abdulsalem, Y. Conway, K Eckler, J. Strategic management of the healthcare supply chain, 2nd ed. Hoboken, NJ: John Wiley & Sons; 2023.

124. Song H, Tucker A, Murrell K. The diseconomies of queue pooling: An empirical investigation of emergency department length of stay. *Manage Sci* 2015; 61(12): 3032–53. https://doi.org/10.1287/mnsc.2014.2118.

125. Senna P, Reis A, Dias A et al. Healthcare supply chain resilience framework: Antecedents, mediators, consequents. *Prod Plann Control* 2023; 34: 295–309. https://doi.org/10.1080/09537287.2021.1913525.

126. Bag S, Gupta S, Choi T-M, Kumar A. Roles of innovation leadership on using big data analytics to establish resilient healthcare supply chains to combat the Covid-19 pandemic: A multimethodological study. *IEEE Trans Eng Manage* 2021; advance online publication 20 August 2021. https://doi.org/10.1109/TEM.2021.3101590.

127. Bohm V, Lacaille D, Spencer N, Barber C. Scoping review of balanced scorecards for use in healthcare settings: Development and implementation. *BMJ Open Qual* 2021; 10(3): 10:e001293. https://doi.org/10.1136/bmjoq-2020-001293

128. Betto F, Sardi A, Garengo P, Sorano E. The evolution of Balanced Scorecard in healthcare: A systematic review of its design, implementation, use and review. *Int J Environ* 2022; 19: 10291. https://doi.org/10.3390/ijerph1916 10291.

129. Teisberg E, Wallace S, O'Hara, S. Defining and implementing value-based health care: A strategic framework. *Acad Med* 2020; 95(5): 682–85. https://doi.org/10.1097/ACM.0000000000003122

130. Ali I, Kannan D. Mapping research on healthcare operations and supply chain management: A topic modelling-based literature review. *Ann Oper Res* 2022; 315: 29–55. https://doi.org/10.1007/s10479-022-04596-5.

131. Jayaraman R, Salah K, King N. Improving opportunities in healthcare supply chain processes via the Internet of Things and Blockchain technology. *Int J Healthc Inf Syst Inform (IJHISI)* 2019; 14: 49–65. https://doi.org/10.4018/IJHISI.2019040104.

132. Aitken J, Esain E, Williams S. Understanding the nature of demand variation of patient arrival for emergency healthcare services. In: Radnor ZJ, Bateman N, Esain A et al., editors. Public service operations management: A research handbook. London: Routledge; 2016: 390–410.

133. Masi D, Day S, Godsell J. Supply chain configurations in the circular economy: A systematic literature review. *Sustainability* 2017; 9: 1602. https://doi.org/10.3390/su9091602.

Gemma Petley

THIS Institute (The Healthcare Improvement Studies Institute)

Gemma is Senior Communications and Editorial Manager at THIS Institute, responsible for overseeing the production and maximising the impact of the series.

Claire Dipple

THIS Institute (The Healthcare Improvement Studies Institute)

Claire is Editorial Project Manager at THIS Institute, responsible for editing and project managing the series.

About the Series

The past decade has seen enormous growth in both activity and research on improvement in healthcare. This series offers a comprehensive and authoritative set of overviews of the different improvement approaches available, exploring the thinking behind them, examining evidence for each approach, and identifying areas of debate.

Cambridge Elements≡

Improving Quality and Safety in Healthcare

Elements in the Series

Collaboration-Based Approaches
Graham Martin and Mary Dixon-Woods

Co-Producing and Co-Designing
Glenn Robert, Louise Locock, Oli Williams, Jocelyn Cornwell,
Sara Donetto and Joanna Goodrich

Implementation Science
Paul Wilson and Roman Kislov

Making Culture Change Happen
Russell Mannion

Operational Research Approaches
Martin Utley, Sonya Crowe and Christina Pagel

Simulation as an Improvement Technique
Victoria Brazil, Eve Purdy and Komal Bajaj

Workplace Conditions
Jill Maben, Jane Ball and Amy C. Edmondson

Governance and Leadership
Naomi J. Fulop and Angus I. G. Ramsay

Health Economics
Andrew Street and Nils Gutacker

Approaches to Spread, Scale-Up, and Sustainability
Chrysanthi Papoutsi, Trisha Greenhalgh and Sonja Marjanovic

Statistical Process Control
Mohammed Amin Mohammed

Values and Ethics
Alan Cribb, Vikki Entwistle and Polly Mitchell

Design Creativity
Gyuchan Thomas Jun, Sue Hignett and P. John Clarkson

Supply Chain Management
Sharon J. Williams

A full series listing is available at: www.cambridge.org/IQ

Printed in the United States
by Baker & Taylor Publisher Services